First Aid Tips
for Parents

by Kate Cronan, M.D.
and Neil Izenberg, M.D.

Burns

Poisoning

Stings
and bites

Head injuries

Seizure or
convulsions and
Heat illness

Broken bones

Bleeding
and wounds

Cold exposure

Eye injuries

Choking

Breathing
emergencies

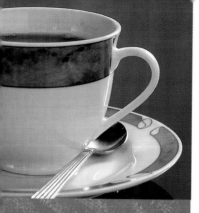

Burns

Preventive measures

- Install a child safety guard on your kitchen stove.

- Don't leave hot liquids unattended.

- Don't drink hot liquids with a child on your lap.

- Check the temperature of the bath water before placing a child in the tub.

- Always supervise children who are in the kitchen during food preparation.

- Install smoke alarms and change the batteries annually.

Most cases of household burns are scald burns which occur when hot liquids are spilled on children, when children touch pots on hot burners or get scalded in a bathtub. Flame burns occur less frequently and result, for example, from pajamas igniting in a house-fire.

The three different degrees of burns are determined by how deep the skin injury is. Second and third degree burns should be treated by a physician.

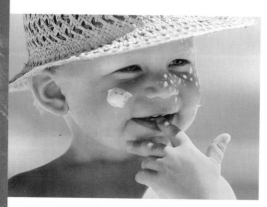

Always apply a sunblock or sunscreen to children who are in the sun!

FIRST-DEGREE

burns are superficial burns, such as sunburn. The skin is dry, red and painful.

SECOND-DEGREE

burns penetrate more deeply into the skin. Water blisters develop and the pain can be severe.

THIRD-DEGREE

burns penetrate to the deepest layers of the skin, causing open sores and some areas of numbness.

What should you do?

If the burn covers a small area of skin:

. Quickly cool the area that has been burned by holding it under lukewarm running water. The water temperature should be about 72 degrees F (i.e., lukewarm, not ice cold). Cooling the area prevents the heat from penetrating more deeply into the skin and reduces the depth of the injury.

2. Give acetaminophen or ibuprofen for pain control appropriate for age and weight. Do not apply home remedies such as butter, ointments, etc.

3. Continue to cool the skin with cool compresses.

If clothes are on fire:

The fire must be extinguished quickly by rolling the child on the ground or smothering the fire with blankets, rugs, etc. Cool the burned area with water; do not remove pieces of clothing that are stuck to the skin.

If there is a large area burned, take your child to the nearest hospital for treatment.

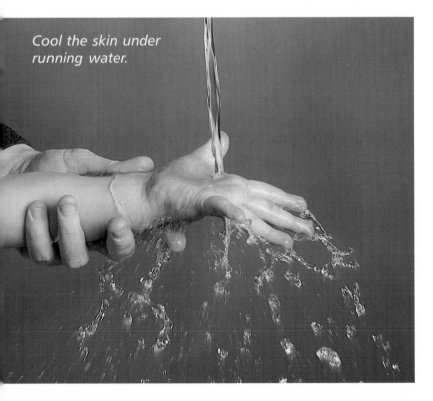

Cool the skin under running water.

911

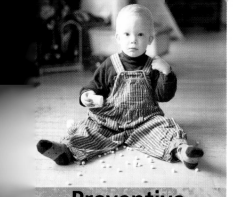

Poisoning

Children can be poisoned by various substances. When a child has been in contact with poisonous substances by swallowing, by skin contact or by inhalation, monitor the child's breathing and level of alertness. Symptoms of poisoning may include nausea, vomiting, cramps, difficulty breathing, unusual odor on breath or unconsciousness. Call your regional poison control center for advice.

Preventive measures

- Store chemicals, detergents, etc. in a safe place out of the reach of children. Make sure that all medicines are kept in a high, locked cabinet.
- Have your regional poison center telephone number posted near the phone.
- Become acquainted with poisonous plants and avoid them in your home.

If a child swallows acids or any other corrosive substance, call poison control center and give the child milk and water to drink.

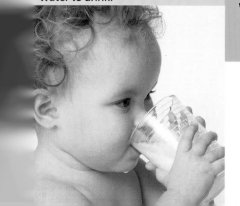

MEDICINES

It may take some time before the poisonous substance is absorbed from the stomach into the bloodstream. Inducing vomiting in order to remove the poison from the stomach may be important in the early phase of poisoning, but this is a decision that should be made by your child's physician and the regional poison control center. Keep Syrup of Ipecac on hand in your home. Small amounts of poisonous substances can lead to life-threatening situations. Even aspirin and acetaminophen can be toxic to a child if large amounts are taken.

What should you do?

Call your regional poison control center for advice. If you need to take your child to the emergency room, take the container of poisonous substance with you.

Corrosive substances

Such as lye, sulfuric acid, nitric acid, acetic acid, caustic soda, liq uid ammonia, ammonium chloride, drain cleaner or automatic dishwasher detergent, as well as gasoline, paint thinner, turpentine, or other petroleum products: Do not induce vomiting as this can burn the throat and esophagus even more. Follow the advice of the poison control center.

Medications, poisonous plants or mushrooms:

Call your regional poison control center.

If the child is already unconscious or lethargic:

1. Call 911.

2. Do not induce vomiting.

3. Do not give the child anything to drink.

4. Keep the airway clear and lay the child on his or her side (see the chapter on Head injuries).

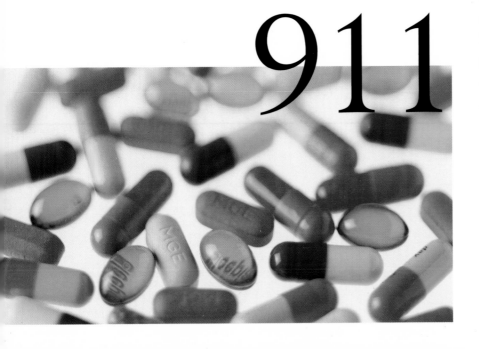

911

If the child is breathing slowly and with difficulty:

1. Call 911.

2. Administer breaths if the child stops breathing (see the chapter on Breathing emergencies).

Skin injuries

Formic acid, pesticides and insecticides, industrial chemicals, acids and lye may cause skin injuries. Some of these substances can penetrate the skin, entering into the body and causing serious poisoning.

1. Call the regional poison control center.

2. Remove clothes which have been soiled by acids or other poisonous liquids.

3. Flood the affected area with water for 10–15 minutes.

Stings and bites

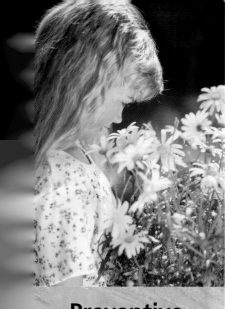

Preventive measures

For insect bites:
- Do not leave juice or other sweet beverages outside in the summer.

- Use insect repellents.

For dog bites:
- Do not allow a child to pet unfamiliar dogs.

- Always supervise young children when they are near dogs.

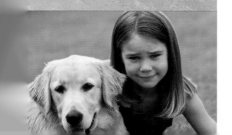

INSECT STINGS

For most children, insect bites cause discomfort, but they are not dangerous. However, some people have strong allergic reactions to specific insect stings or bites and can go into shock.

DANGER SIGNS

Pale, cold or clammy skin. Trouble breathing or wheezing; a feeling of throat tightening; a rapid pulse, which may be difficult to find (often higher than 140); semi-consciousness.

REPELLENTS

A repellent containing no more than a 10% concentration of DEET should be selected. Use sparingly on young children and not at all on infants. Follow the label directions carefully. Do not apply over cuts or irritated skin, or hands, near eyes and mouth or under clothing. After returning indoors, wash treated skin with soap and water. If you prefer a non-chemical repellent, any product containing citronella will work. You should not allow your child to apply repellents.

911

What should you do?

Insect stings

To relieve discomfort, apply a cool wet cloth or ice to the insect bite area. If itching and swelling persist, you may use Benadryl. Check package for appropriate dosing. If rash develops and spreads, contact your doctor. If the child becomes pale, gets clammy skin, develops a rapid pulse rate or shows signs of semiconsciousness or breathing trouble:

1. Call 911.

2. Begin rescue breathing if the child stops breathing (see chapter on Breathing emergencies).

Dog bites

If a dog bite penetrates the skin, stitches may be needed. Contact your child's physician for advice. Within a few days the bite may, in rare circumstances, cause a skin infection. Contact a physician.

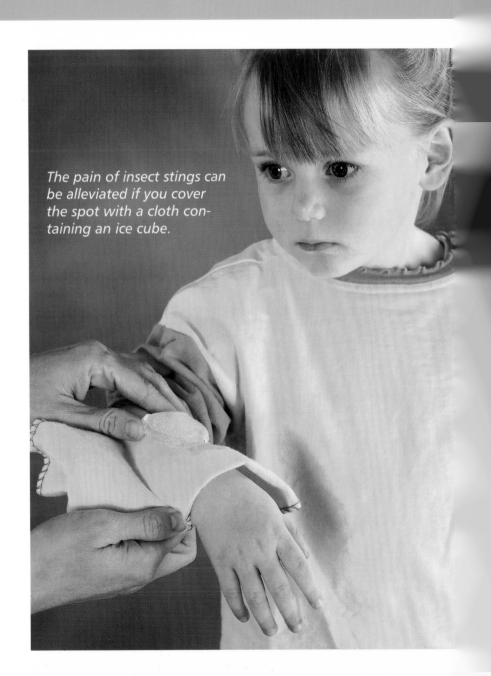

The pain of insect stings can be alleviated if you cover the spot with a cloth containing an ice cube.

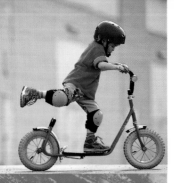

Preventive measures

To avoid head injuries:

- Children should always wear helmets and other protective gear when biking, skating, or skateboarding.

- Make sure that shelves and cupboards are fastened to the wall, so they will not fall on a child who might be climbing them.

- Install gates at the doorways of bedrooms.

- Open second story screens from the top only.

- Avoid the use of trampolines at all times.

Head injuries

Children most often incur head injuries from a fall. Many head injuries result in facial wounds or scalp wounds. Such wounds often bleed profusely at first. If the cut appears to be gaping, contact your child's physician.

If the child falls or receives a blow to the head, it is possible that an internal injury occurred. It is important to note whether the child loses consciousness. The child may appear pale and clammy at first. Your child will probably become sleepy after the fall and it is not a problem for the child to sleep as long as he/she can be easily aroused again.

It is not unusual for a child to vomit after a head injury. If the child vomits many times, it could be a reason for concern. This could be anything from a simple concussion to bleeding inside the skull.

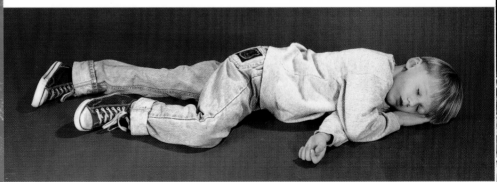

Lay the child on his or her side, with the top leg bent at the hip and the knee resting on the floor. Bend the top arm and place the child's hand under his or her head. Stretch out the lower arm in front of the body.

What should you do?

Head injuries that are bleeding:

1. Bring the edges of the wound together with a bandage or hold a compress against the scalp.

2. Apply pressure until the bleeding stops. You may use a cap to hold the compress in place.

3. Contact the child's physician.

Bleeding from inside the ear:

1. Contact your child's physician.

2. Place a loose bandage on the outer ear. Do not insert anything into the ear canal.

If the child is unconscious or increasingly sleepy:

1. Call 911.

2. Monitor the child's breathing. The neck may be injured. You should not move the child until trained help arrives unless not moving the child will cause life-threatening harm.

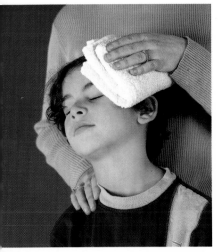

Bring the edges of the wound together and apply a compress, such as a towel, to the wound.

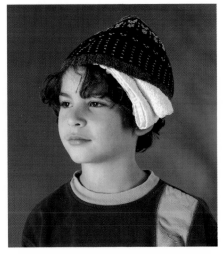

Use a cap to hold the compress tightly in place.

911

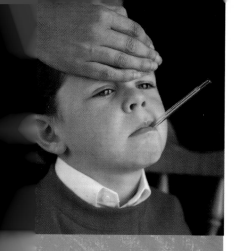

Seizure or convulsions

Children may have seizures or convulsions which can be due to high fever or other causes such as infection, injury or a seizure disorder. If a child has a seizure, the reason may not be clear until the child has been seen or treated by a physician. If a seizure begins and lasts for more than five minutes, or if the child turns blue, call 911. Make sure that the child's airway is open and that he/she is breathing (refer to Breathing emergencies chapter). Do not give the child any medicine by mouth.

Preventive measures

Heat illness
- Remove blankets and warm clothes when body temperature exceeds 100 degrees F.

- Avoid vigorous exercise if the temperature is extremely high.

- Remember to give the child plenty to drink.

Heat illnesses

Symptoms of heat exhaustion are fatigue, nausea, dizziness, thirst, or confusion. This occurs in extremely hot weather during strenuous physical exertion. Heat stroke is more serious and the symptoms are: absence of sweating, hot, flushed skin, muscle cramps, nausea, vomiting, and rapid pulse.

911

What should you do?

Convulsions

1. If your child is having convulsions, do not move or restrain the child.

2. Move objects out of the way to prevent injury.

3. Loosen clothing.

4. Gently turn the child's head to one side to keep the airway open and clear.

5. Call your doctor after the seizure to discuss next steps.

Children who have convulsions should be examined by a physician as a matter of precaution. Call 911 if the seizure continues for more than five minutes or if the child is turning blue.

Heat illness

1. If your child has heat exhaustion, cool your child by moistening his or her clothing with cold water.

2. Call your child's physician if the child is not responding to the above treatment. If you suspect heat stroke, call 911.

3. Give your child plenty to drink if he/she is conscious and awake.

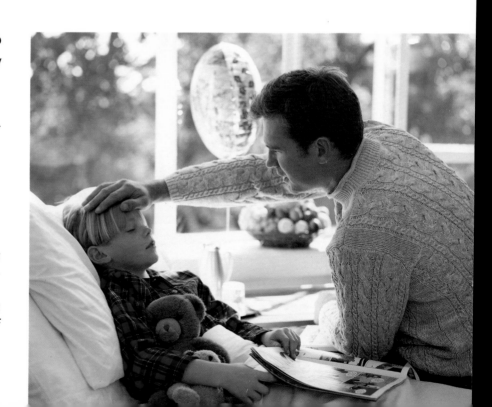

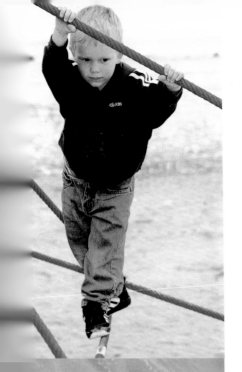

Broken bones

Signs of broken bones include pain, dislocation, unnatural mobility, or an arm or leg that appears shorter than usual. Swelling in the area of a bone or joint after an injury may also suggest a fracture. In the event of a fracture or suspected fracture, the child must be examined by a physician.

Preventive measures

Dislocated elbow:

- Avoid pulling a child's arm vigorously when you are in a hurry or when lifting the child. Stop and wait, or lift the child by placing your hands under both armpits.

Broken bones:

- Always supervise a young child during play and outdoor activities. Prevent children from standing in grocery carts, and on chairs and tables.

BROKEN RIBS

Ribs can be broken by falling or by blows to the chest. The child will experience sharp pain, particularly when breathing deeply or coughing. There is no appropriate first aid, but exertion should be avoided. The child should be seen by a doctor if there is a concern for rib fractures, especially if there is trouble breathing.

DISLOCATED ELBOW

If a child's arm is jerked hard (i.e. if you help a child who is falling or who must be lifted up), one of the elbow bones can become dislocated. This happens to infants and toddlers up to the age of 4 years. A dislocated elbow is painful; the child will cry and will resist moving his or her elbow. Contact a physician and explain exactly what happened, as this type of injury can rarely be seen on an X-ray.

What should you do?

Broken ankle, thigh, shin or foot:

1. Support the leg by rolling up a blanket on each side of the leg. Place padding under the knee.

2. If the child must be carried to a place where emergency medical caregivers can take over, a soft splint should be applied. Gently wrap a soft object (a folded blanket or pillow) around the injured area. Fasten it to the leg with wide scarves or strips of cloth to reduce mobility in joints above and below the fracture.

911

Please note! Do not tie the healthy leg to the injured leg, as normal movement in the healthy leg will jar the injured leg.

Broken arm or hand

1. Do not move the injured body part.

2. The joints above and below the fractured arm should not be moved. This reduces the pain and risk of complications. If the fracture is accompanied by an open wound, the wound must be covered. If bone fragments are protruding from the wound, first wrap something around them so that they are not pressed into the wound when you bandage it.

If you suspect a fracture in the collarbone, shoulder, upper or lower arm, hand or fingers, place the arm in a sling.

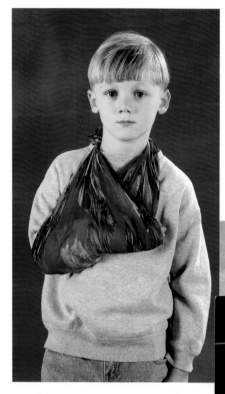

In the event of a suspected fracture, place the arm in a simple temporary sling. Use whatever you have at hand – a shawl, a scarf, etc. The child's hand should be raised to about 4 inches above the elbow and fingertips should be exposed. Knot should be tied at the side of the neck opposite the injury. Place a pad under the knot.

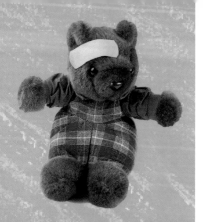

Bleeding and wounds

Preventive measures

- Travel with a simple first aid kit (containing bandages, disinfectant and adhesive strips).

- Avoid situations where young children are at risk of falling.

- Provide careful supervision when young children are playing inside and outdoors.

- To prevent falls: keep children away from stairs until they are capable of getting up and down.

VISIBLE BLEEDING

Bleeding from arteries is bright red and occurs in spurts. Bleeding from veins flows more smoothly and is dark-colored.

INTERNAL BLEEDING

There may be bleeding inside the body following a fracture or injury to internal organs. There is reason to suspect internal bleeding if the child has suffered a blow to the chest or abdomen and complains of pain, has difficulty breathing, has a rapid pulse rate, is pale or lightheaded. When an arm or leg is crushed or a thigh or hip is fractured, there may also be severe internal bleeding.

911

What should you do?

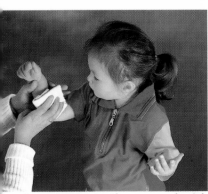

Apply pressure to the wound with clean, dry dressings.

Wounds

Cuts (lacerations)

. Call 911 if a limb or body part is detached or if internal bleeding is suspected.

. Apply pressure to the wound with clean, dry dressings. If the dressings soak through, layer a new dressing on top. Do not remove soaked dressing as this will restart bleeding.

. Elevate the part of the body that is bleeding.

. If the cut continues to bleed or if it is gaping, take your child to a physician.

5. If a limb or body part is detached, firmly bandage the stump. The detached part should be placed in a clean plastic bag and transported with the child to an emergency room.

Scrapes and abrasions

Wash gently with soap and water. Cover with a clean bandage. If the abrasion is very large or there is dirt or gravel, or if glass is suspected to be in the wound, contact your child's physician.

Puncture wounds

These can occur from knives or nails and usually do little damage to the skin, but there may be deeper injuries. There is often contamination, which may cause infection deep in the wound. Contact your child's physician.

Contusions

These are bruises caused by blunt injury. They can be minor or serious depending upon the impact and the location on the body. Contact your child's physician if the contusions appear to be large or over important structures such as the abdomen, chest or face.

Nose bleeds

1. If your child's nose begins to bleed and continues, apply pressure across the lower part of the nose by pinching and continue this for at least 5 minutes. The child should be seated.

2. If the bleeding continues after this has been done, call the child's physician or go to the emergency room.

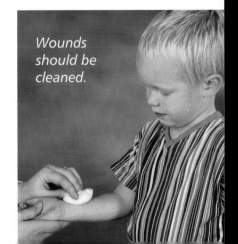

Wounds should be cleaned.

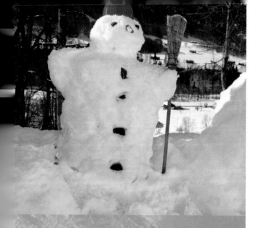

Cold exposure

Preventive measures

- Have your child dress warmly when going outside in cold temperatures.

- A windproof outer layer of clothing protects against the wind.

- In cold weather, keep the child's clothing dry at all times.

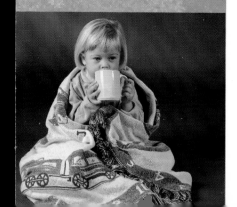

DEEP FROSTBITE

The frostbite may penetrate more deeply. The skin may change color and become dark.

SUPERFICIAL FROSTBITE

Fingers, toes, ears, nose and cheeks are most likely to be affected. The skin becomes stiff, there is a ting-ling sensation followed by numb-ness. White patches become visi-ble on the skin.

HYPOTHERMIA

After prolonged exposure to cold often combined with wind, the temperature of the entire body may drop. Your child may have shivering, weakness, confusion and drowsiness.

What should you do

Deep frostbite

If you suspect that the frostbite is deep, take the child indoors, wrap the affected areas and call your child's doctor immediately.

Superficial frostbite

Take your child indoors. Place the frostbitten area in warm water for 20 to 30 minutes.

Hypothermia

1. Take your child indoors imme-diately. Remove wet clothes.

2. Wrap in warm blankets. Deter-mine if your child is conscious.

3. If the child is conscious, give him or her a warm drink.

4. Call your child's physician.

Eye injuries

Accidental chemical exposures to the eye can result in burns to the eye. Children can get poked in the eye with objects such as pencils, sticks, etc. This can result in serious eye injuries or scratches to the surface of the eye.

What should you do?

For chemical exposures

. Flood the eye with generous amounts of lukewarm water.

. Call your regional poison control center for further advice.

911

Other eye injuries

1. If a child's eye is scraped, contact your child's physician. If an object such as a pencil is poked in the eye, have your child seen by a medical professional. An eye doctor may be needed.

2. Do not put any drops in the child's eye. If the area around the eye is bleeding, apply gentle pressure until the bleeding stops and seek medical attention.

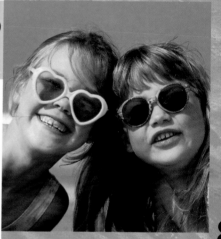

Children who are outdoors in bright sunlight should wear sunglasses to protect their eyes. On snowy mountains, it is important to wear sunglasses both on sunny days and when the sky is overcast.

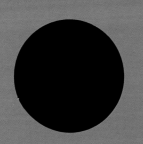

Do not let a child play with toys or small items that can fit through this hole. Small objects can cause the child to choke.

Preventive measures

- Inspect the child's toys and remove any that have small parts that are loose or may loosen.

- Be attentive when introducing solid foods. Avoid foods such as popcorn, peanuts, grapes, carrots, small hard candy and hot dog chunks until the age of four.

- Always provide supervision when young children are eating or playing with toys.

Choking

Children often put things in their mouths when exploring their environment. Small objects can get stuck in the windpipe and cause choking. Choking may also occur when the child makes the transition from liquids and mashed foods to solid foods. When a child is choking, the windpipe is partially or fully blocked. The child becomes frightened and the face turns a grayish blue. The child may then lose consciousness. Choking can be life-threatening, and a quick response is needed. For children under four years, many foods and objects are dangerous.

SWALLOWED FOREIGN OBJECTS

If a child swallows a button, coin, etc., this is seldom serious. These objects are passed into the stomach and eliminated on their own. If the child swallows a sharp object such as a piece of glass, needle, etc., you should call your child's physician.

FOREIGN OBJECTS IN THE EARS/NOSE

Small children may also put objects in their ear canals or in their noses. Try to remove the object only if it is close to the edge of the ear canal or nostril. Contact a physician for advice if you cannot easily remove the object.

911